ISBN-10: 0615576591
ISBN-13: 978-0615576596 (Little Vet)

For more information visit us at www.LittleVet.com

Disclaimer: This book should not be used to diagnose
or treat any medical condition in animals.

Mavis the Rescued Tortoise

A Little Vet™ Book

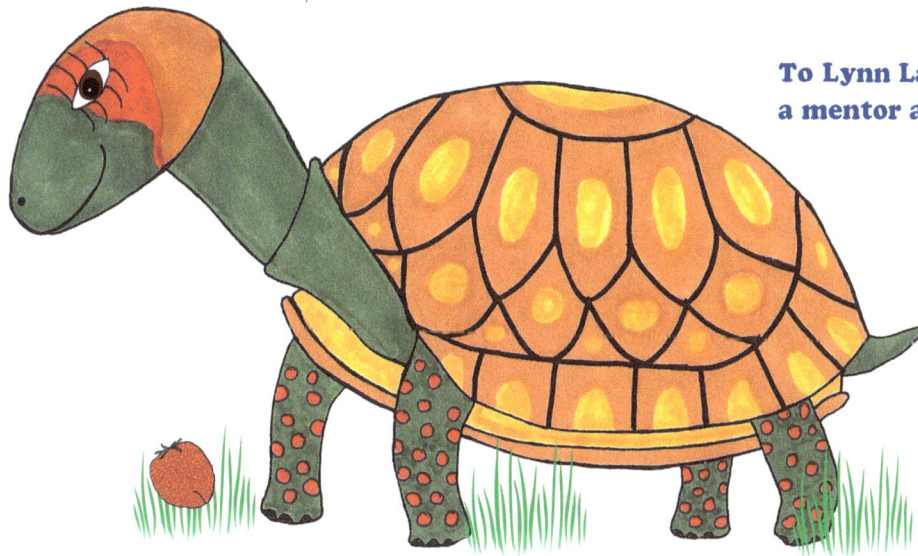

To Lynn Lawhon, DVM,
a mentor and friend

Story by: Lori J. Hehn, DVM
Pictures by: Don E. Winters

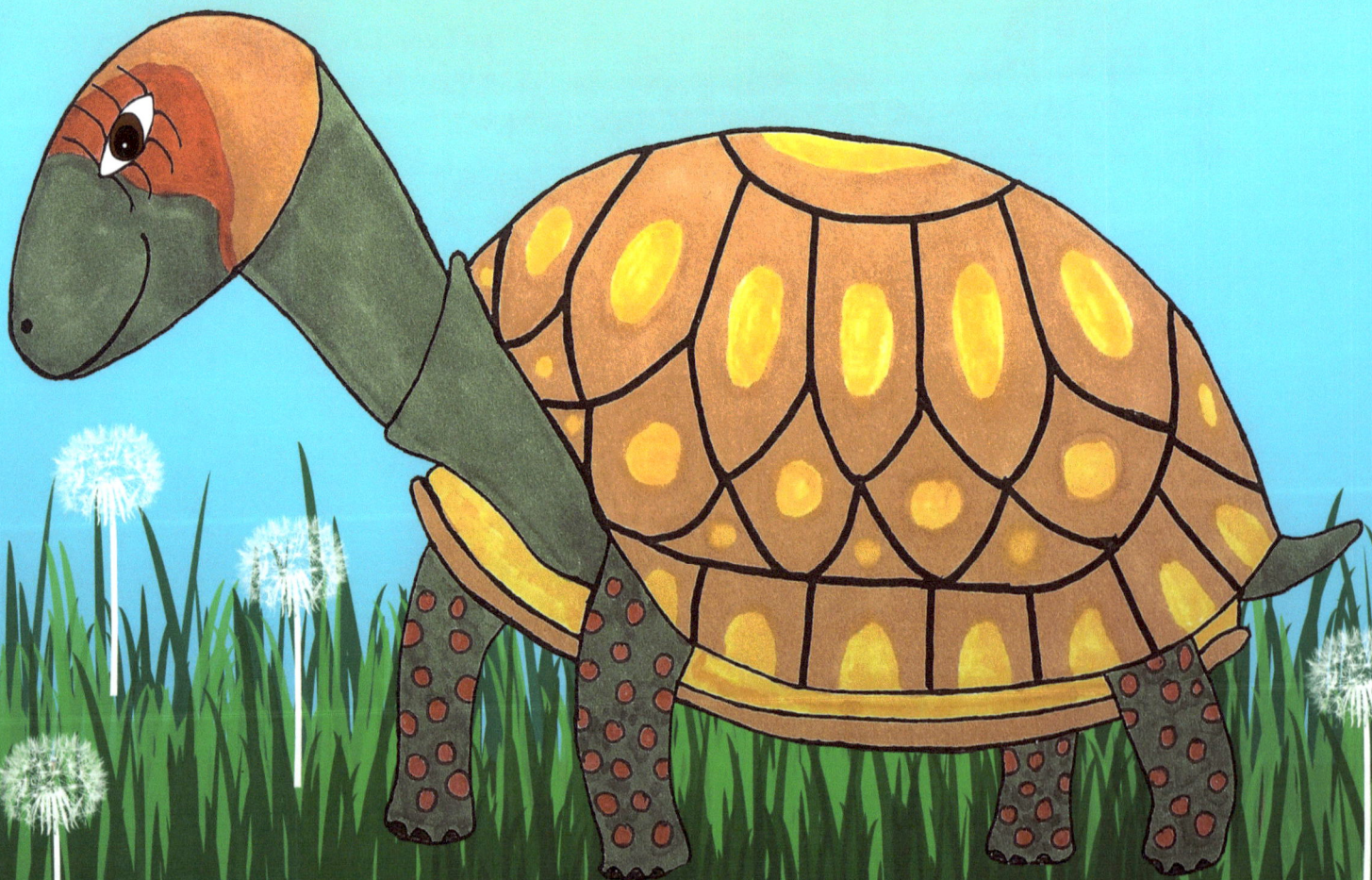

This is my pet tortoise Mavis Maribelle Mayflower. She is a very unique tortoise because she has a flower on her shell. That is how she got her name!

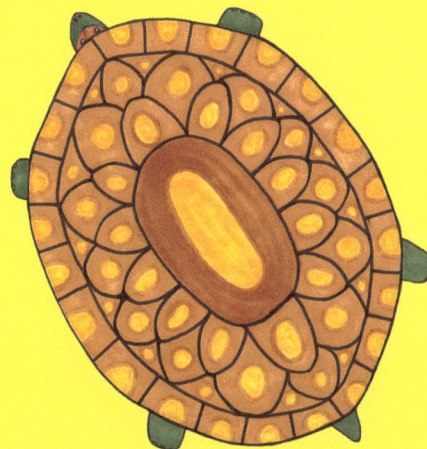

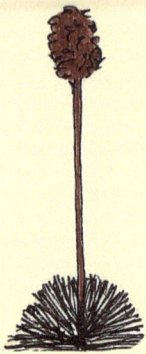

My dad taught me the difference between a tortoise and a turtle.

A tortoise lives mostly on land, while a turtle lives mostly in the water.

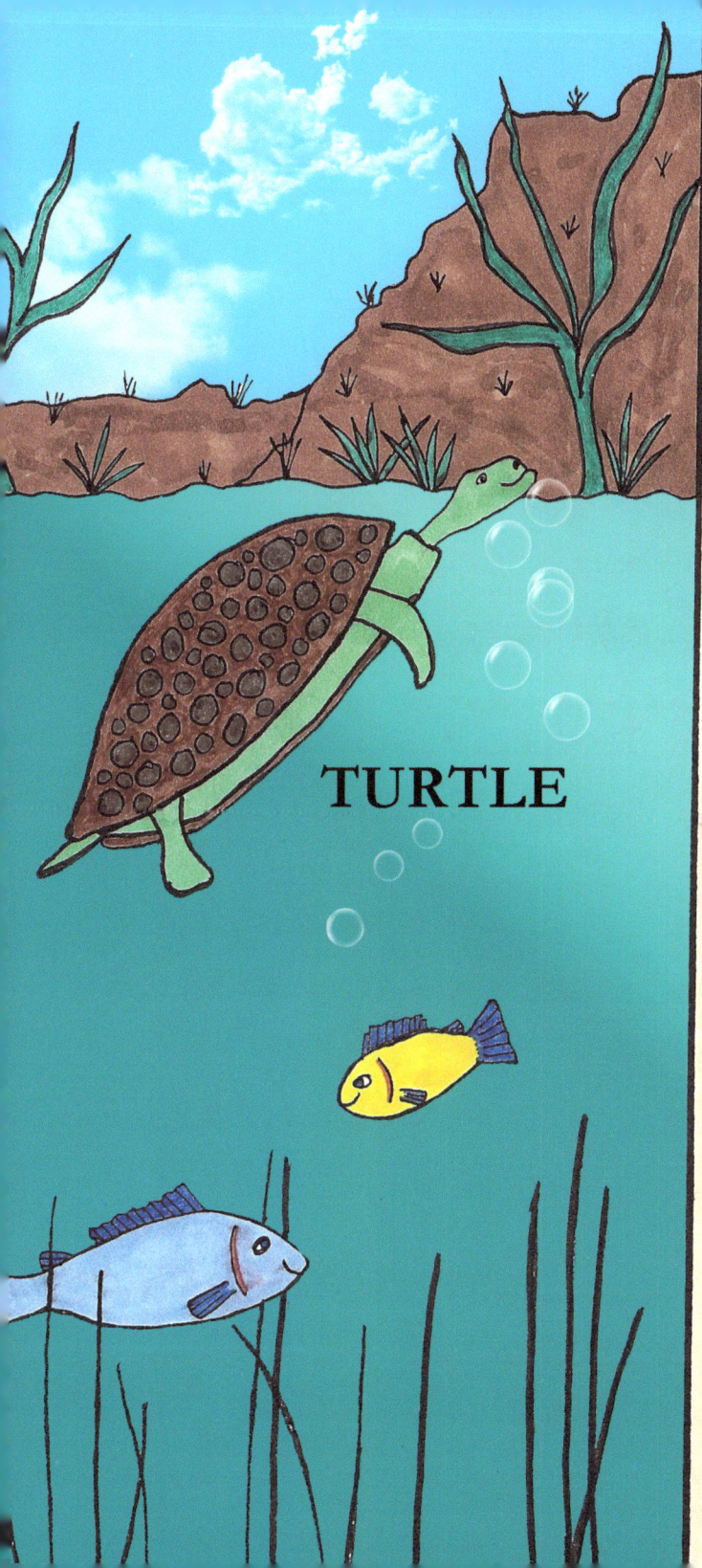

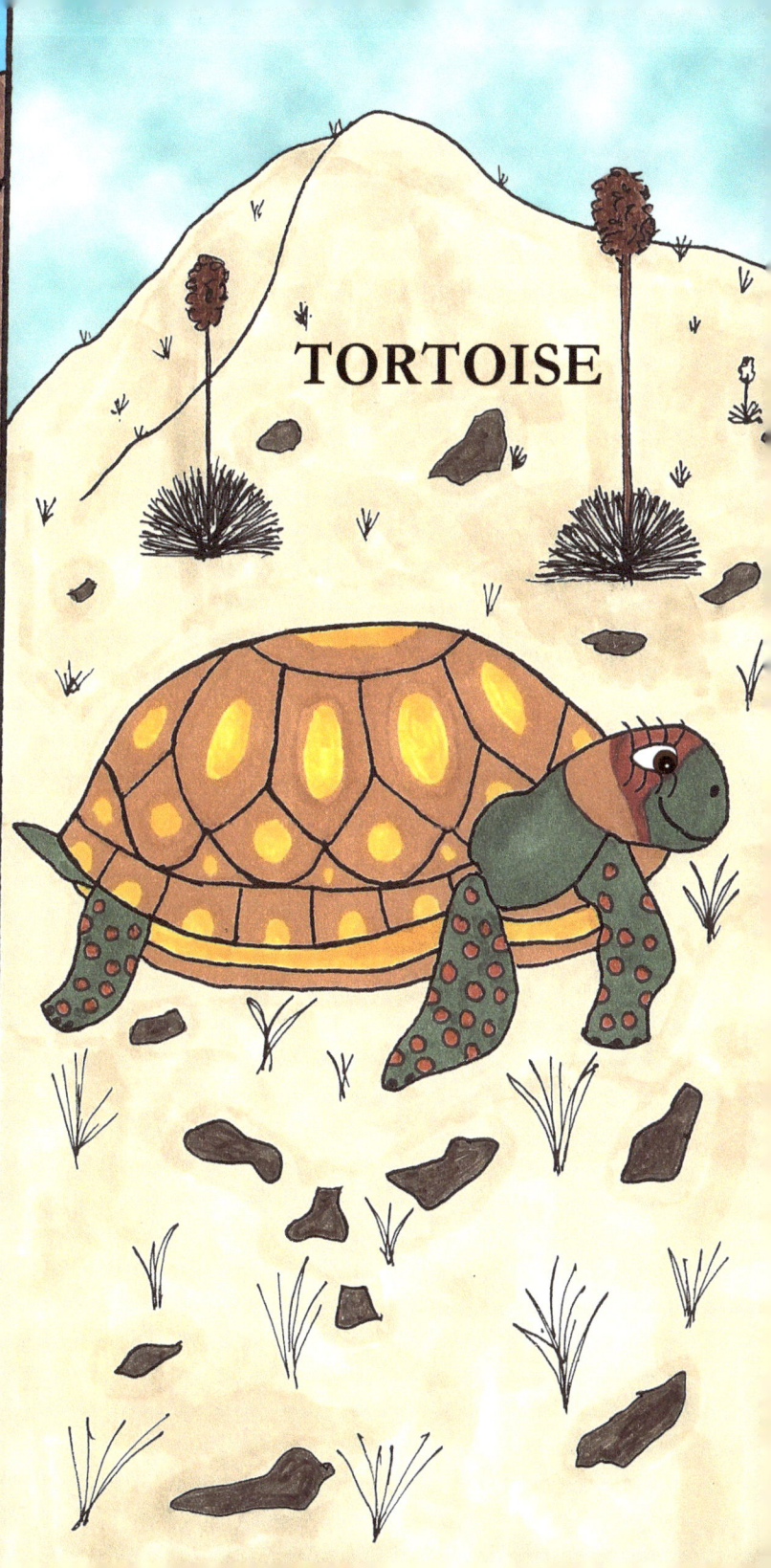

TURTLE

TORTOISE

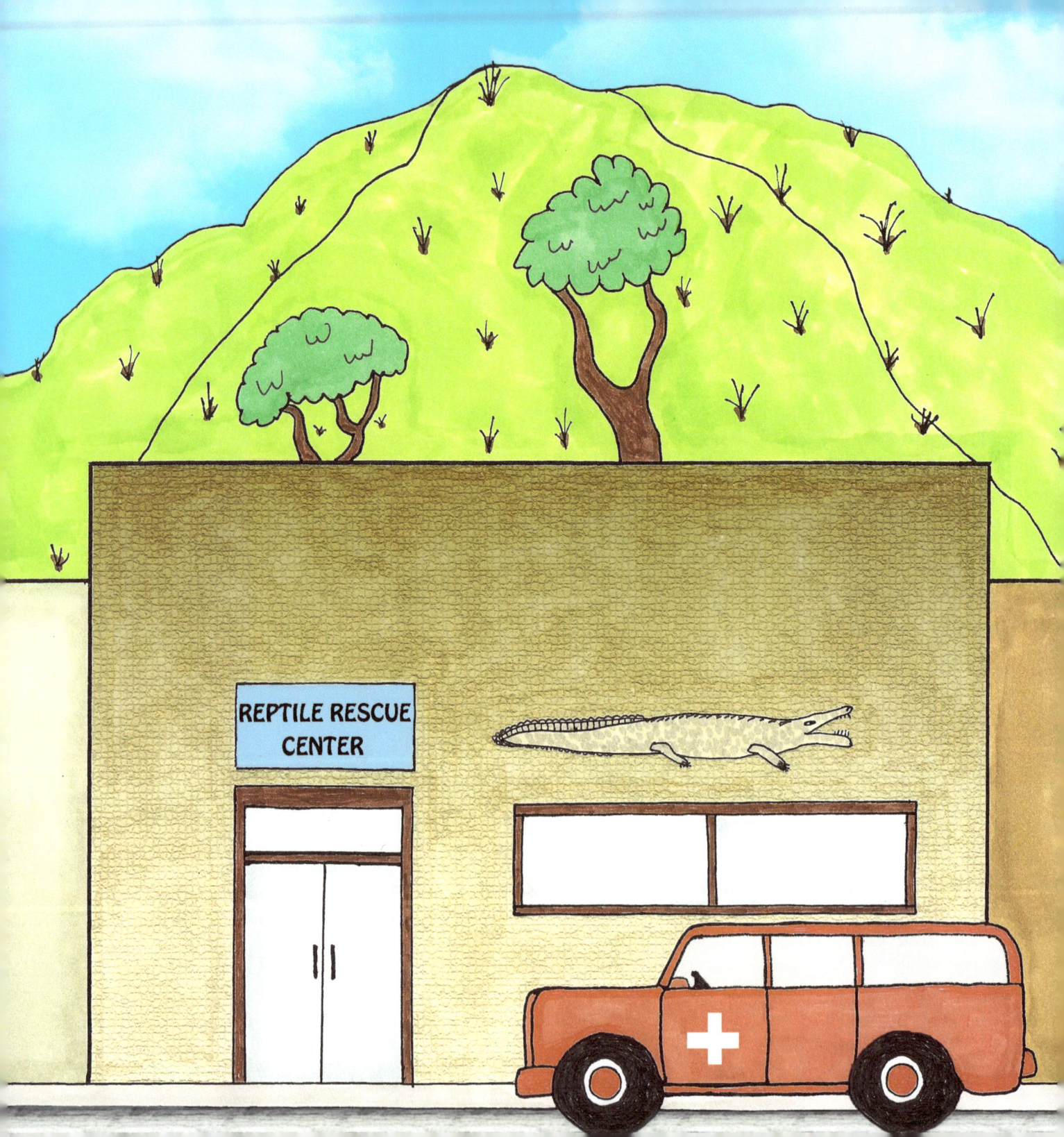

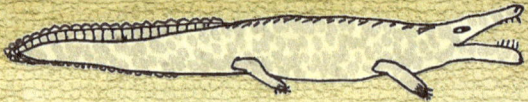

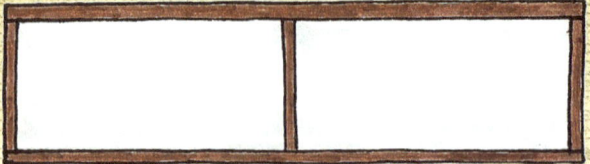

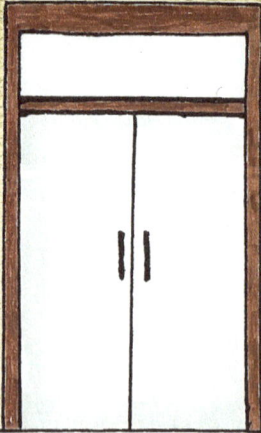

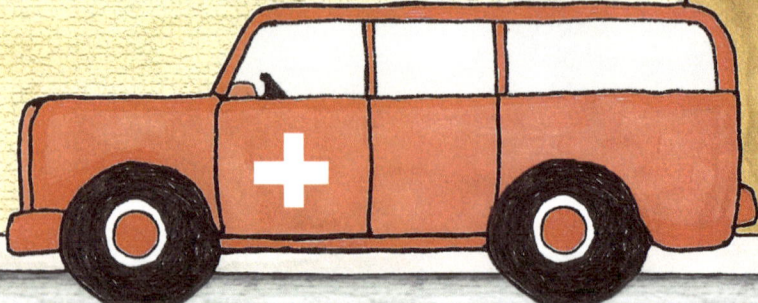

Mavis was brought to the Reptile Rescue Center last May because she was found injured in a drainage ditch, and she couldn't climb out on her own!

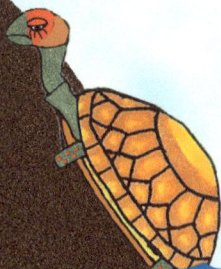

The exotics veterinarian said she is a red footed tortoise and a rare breed. I think she is beautiful! They are originally from South America. She may live up to 50 years, or even longer, if we take great care of her!

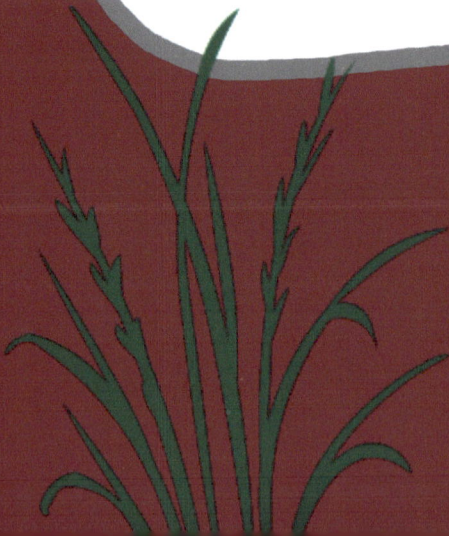

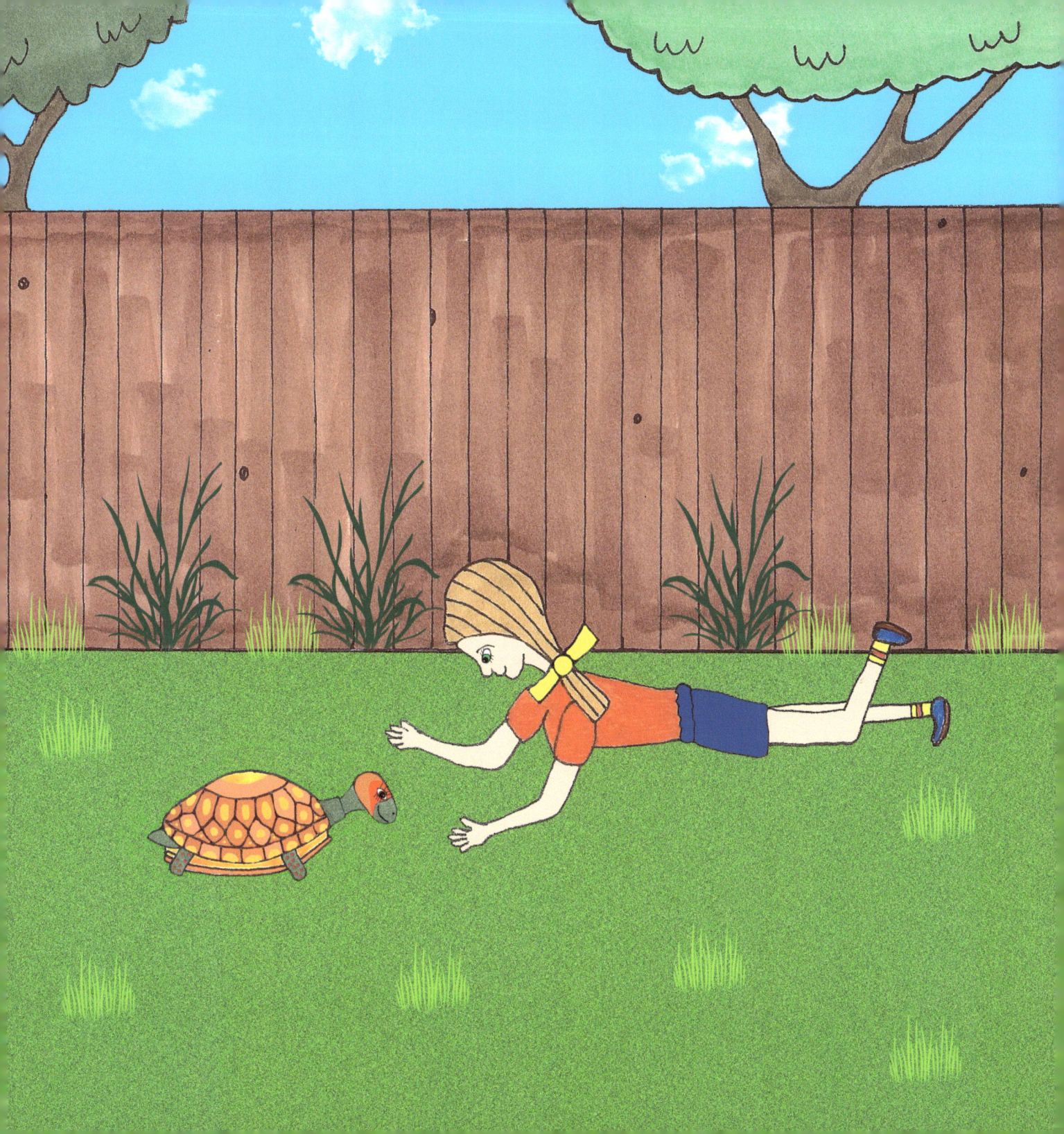

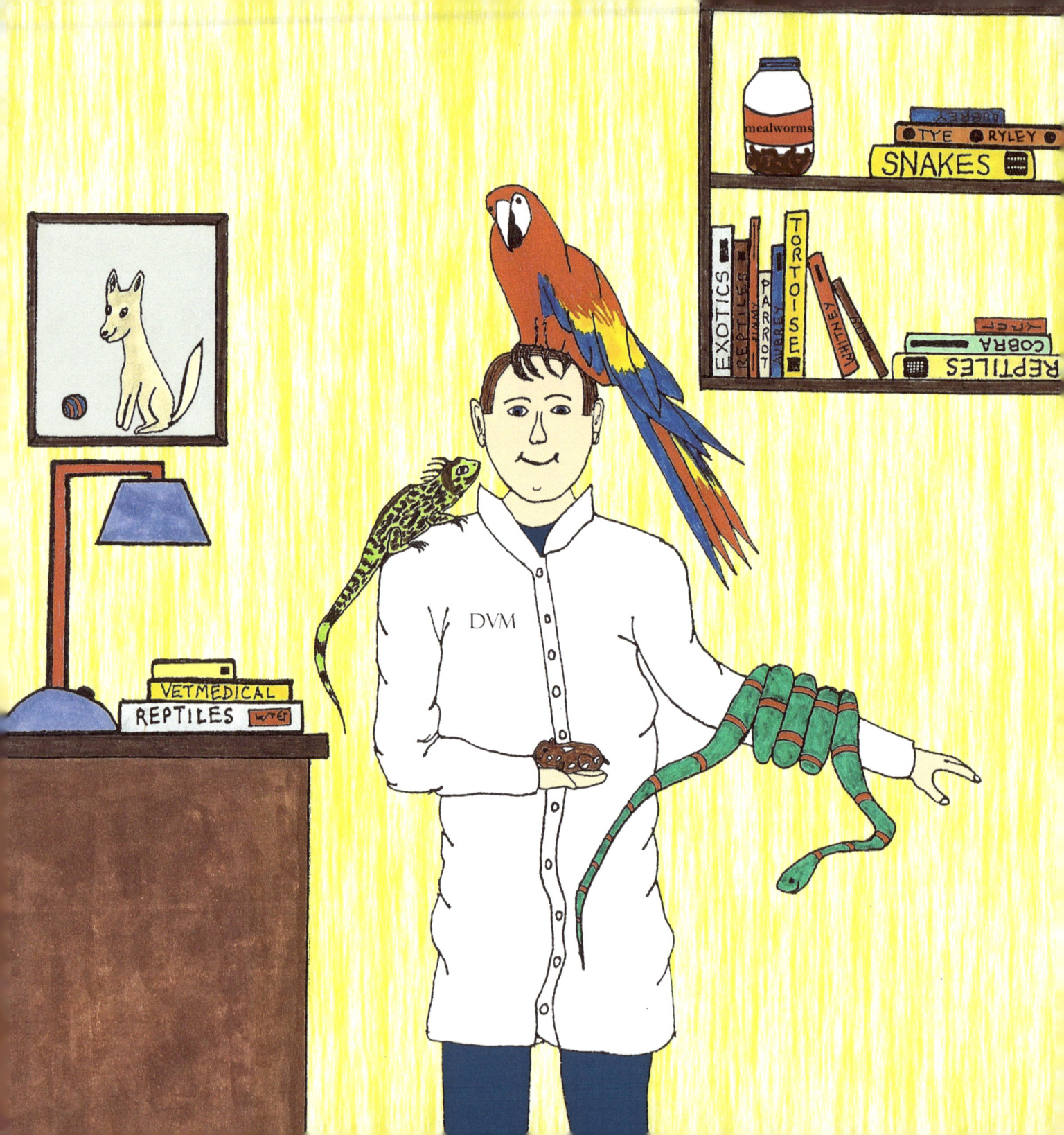

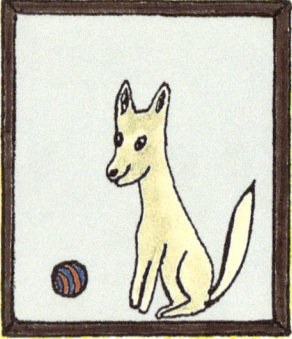

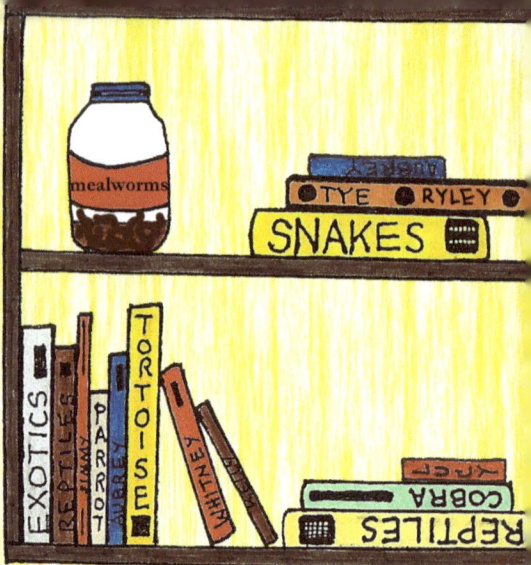

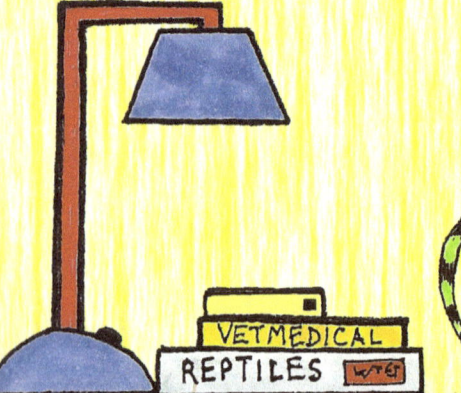

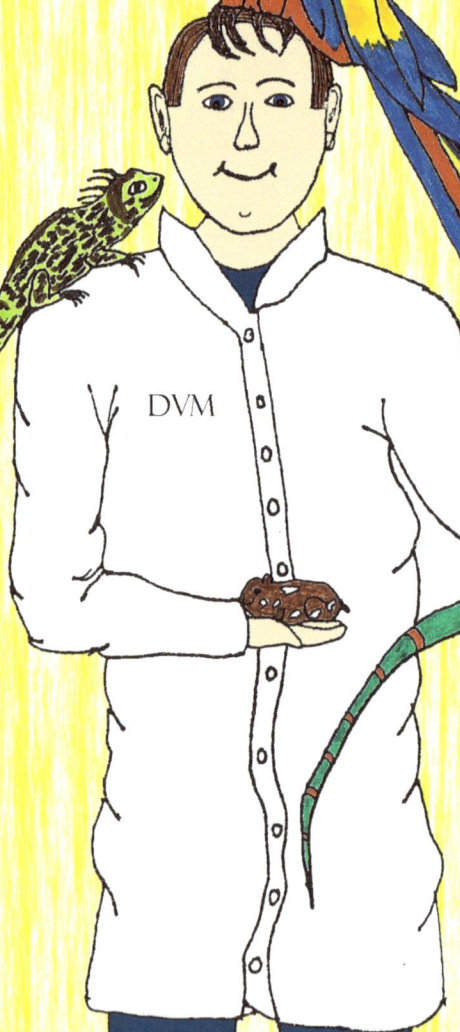

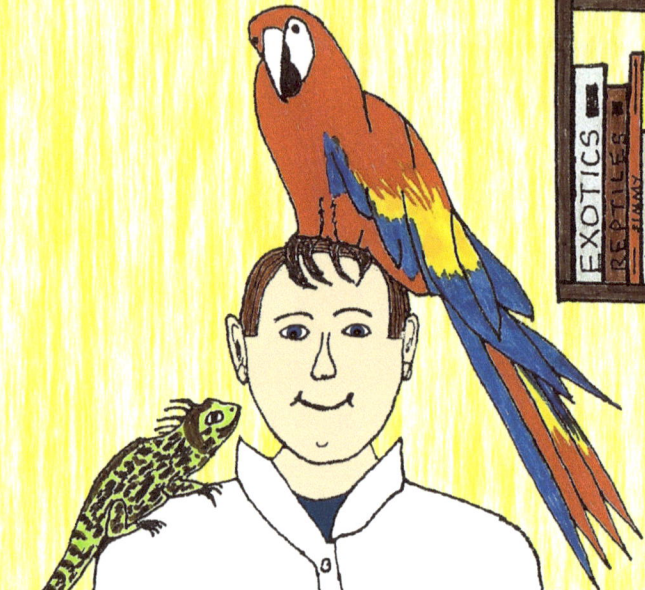

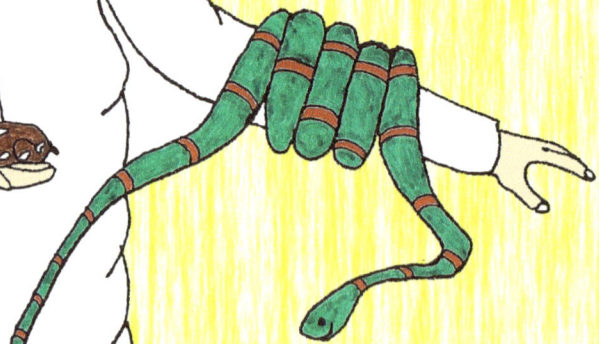

An exotics vet is a doctor who treats exotic animals like birds, reptiles, hamsters, and other unique creatures.

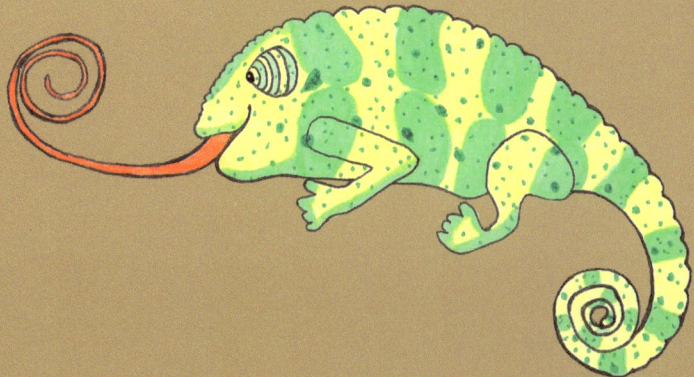

When Mavis came to the Reptile Rescue Center, she was dehydrated and needed some special care.

She made some new tortoise friends while she was there!

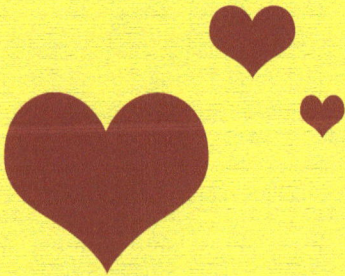

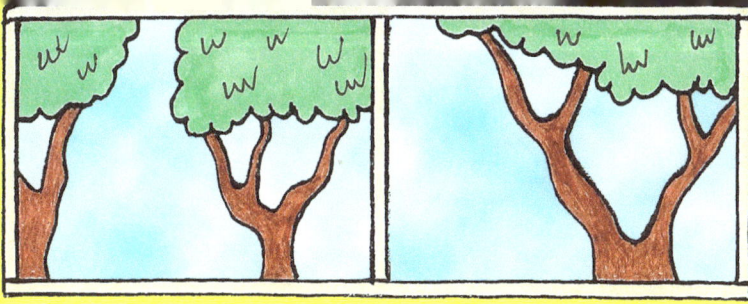

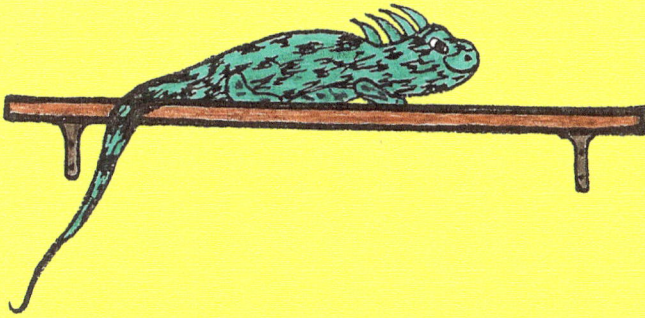

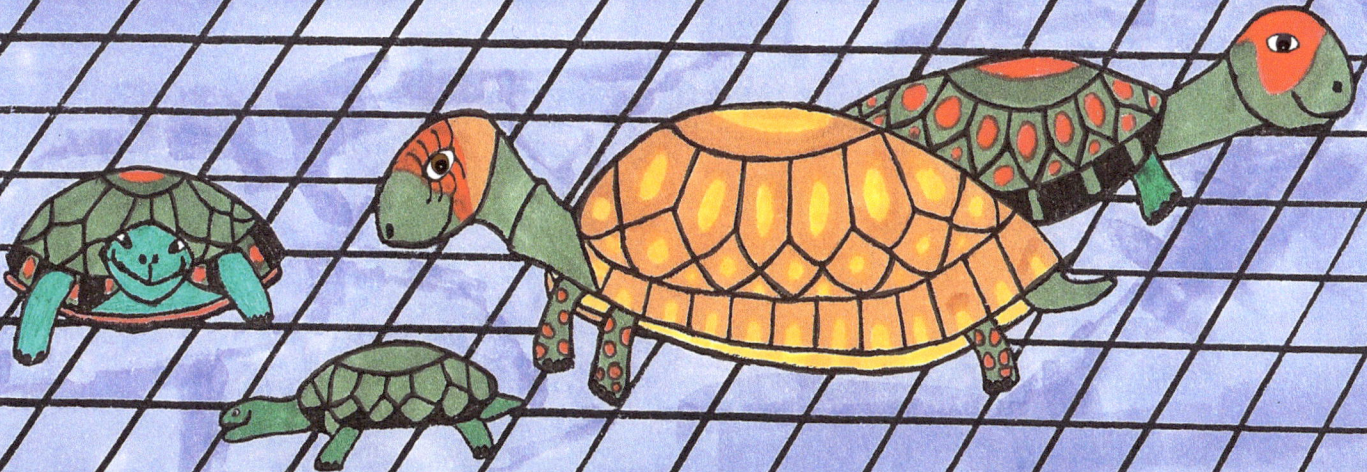

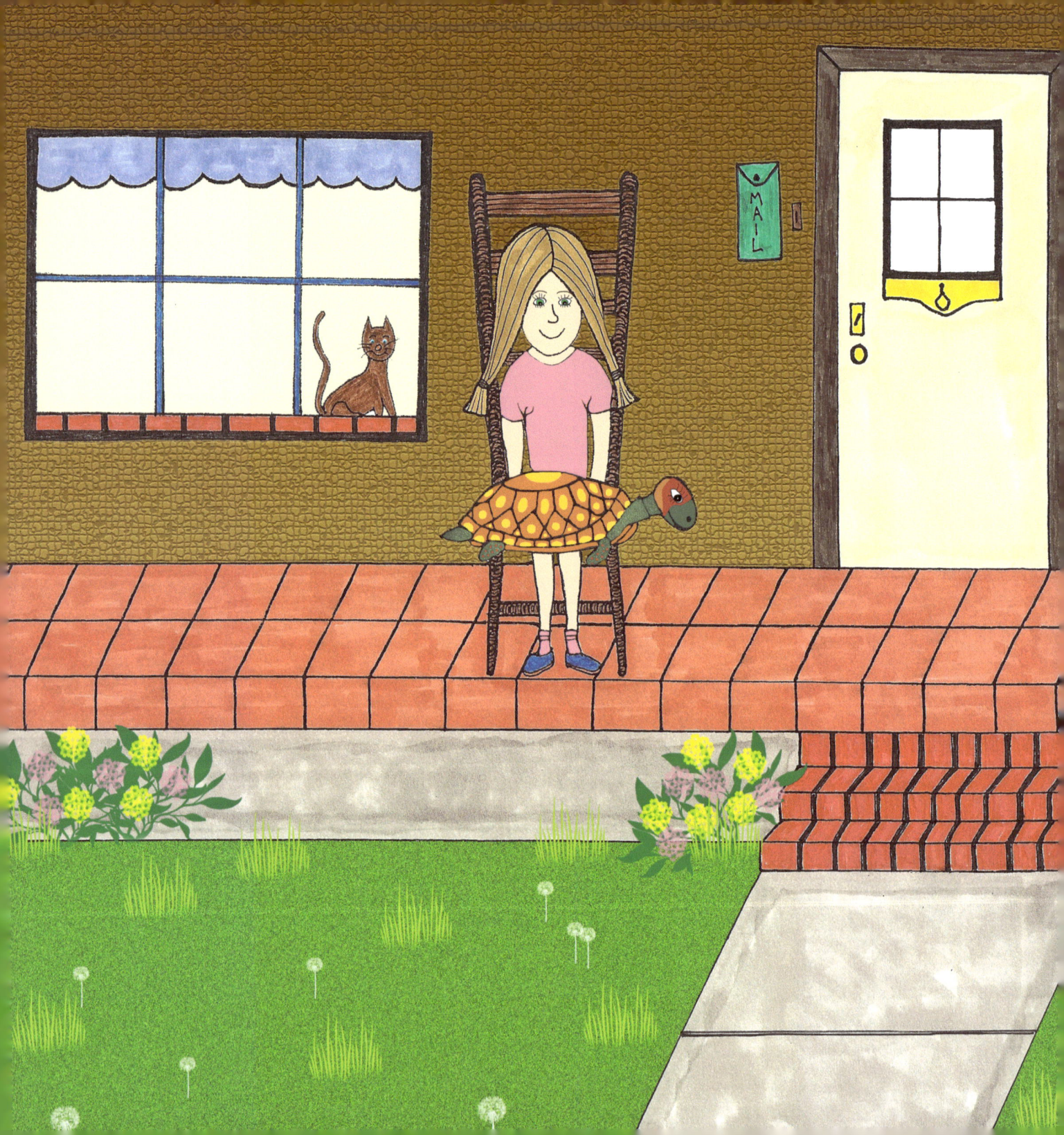

After she was well, my dad brought her home to be our pet. She is very friendly, and after I play with her I have to wash my hands.

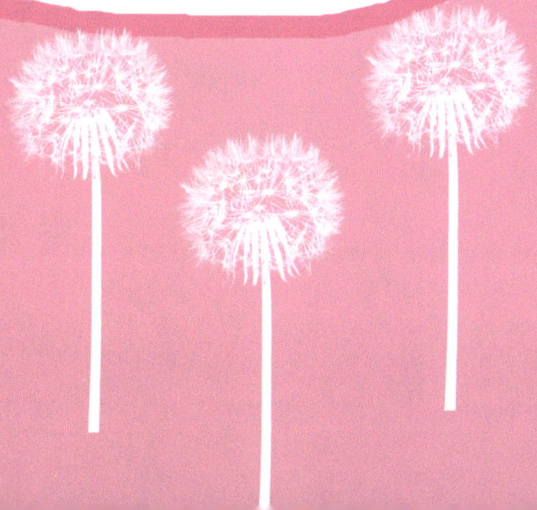

My dad is a herpetologist who works at the center. A herpetologist is a scientist who studies reptiles!

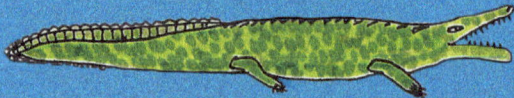

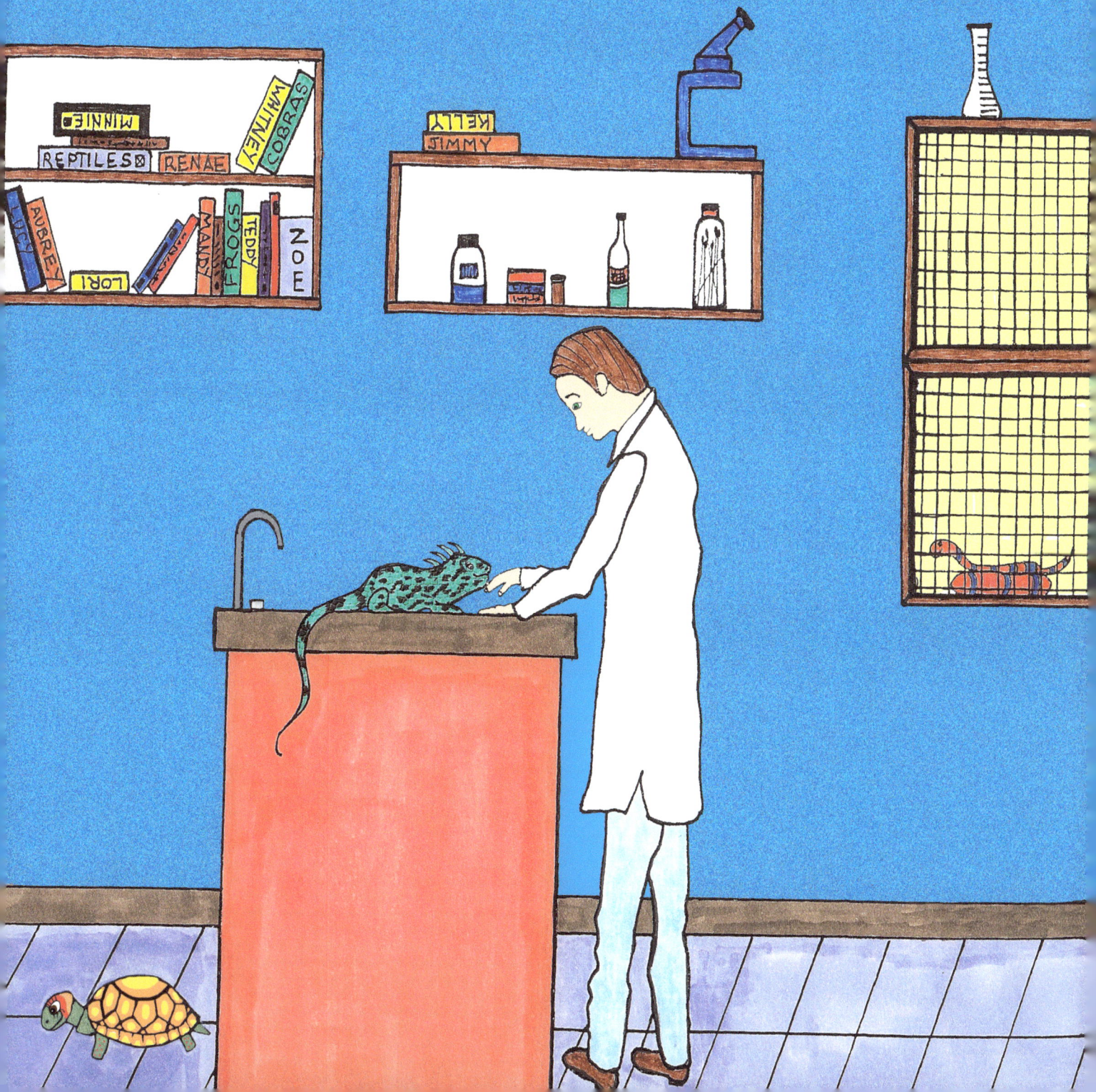

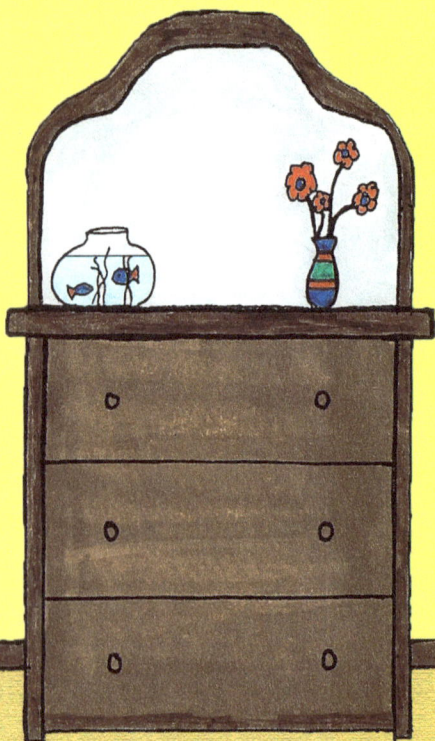

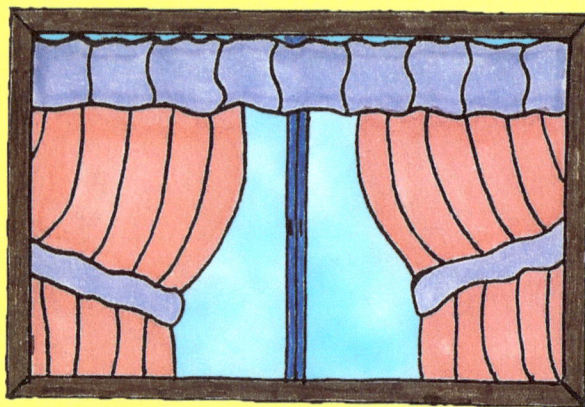

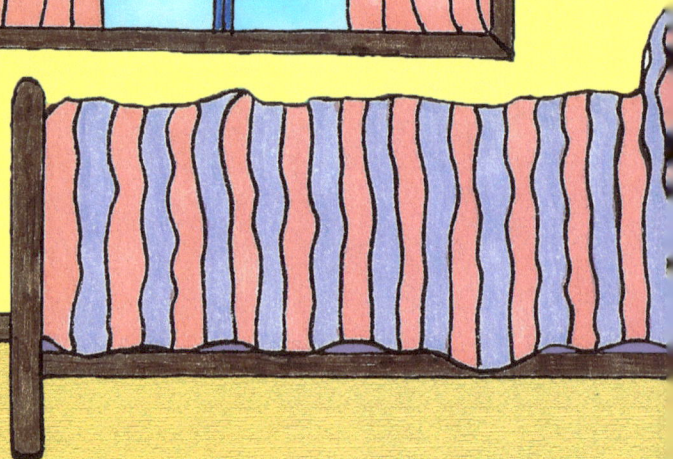

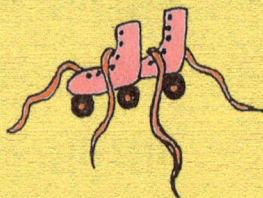

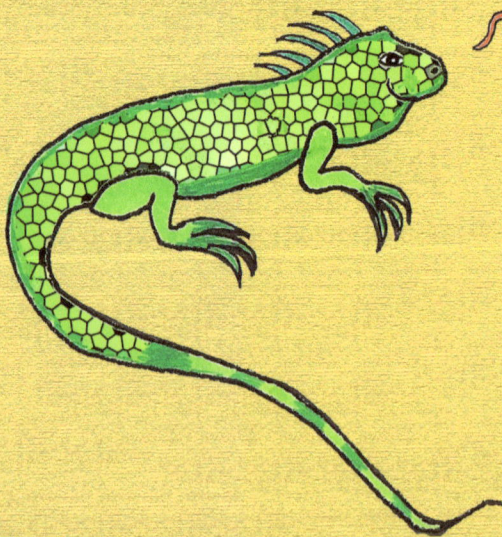

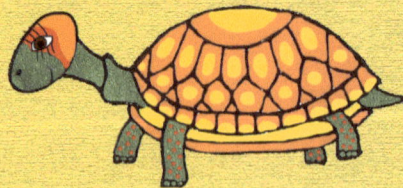

We also have a pet iguana and a pet snake at my house. They like Mavis!

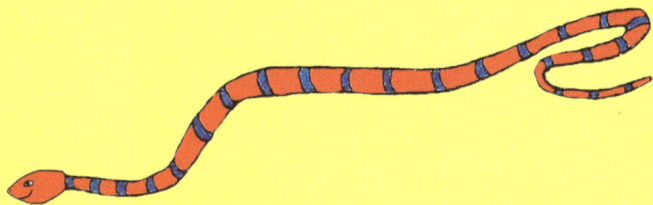

Reptiles like Mavis require a very special habitat so they can stay healthy. They need to have a place with the perfect temperature and humidity.

Mavis loves to spend time in her terrarium!

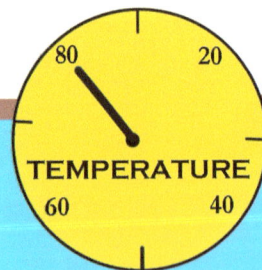

TEMPERATURE
80 20
60 40

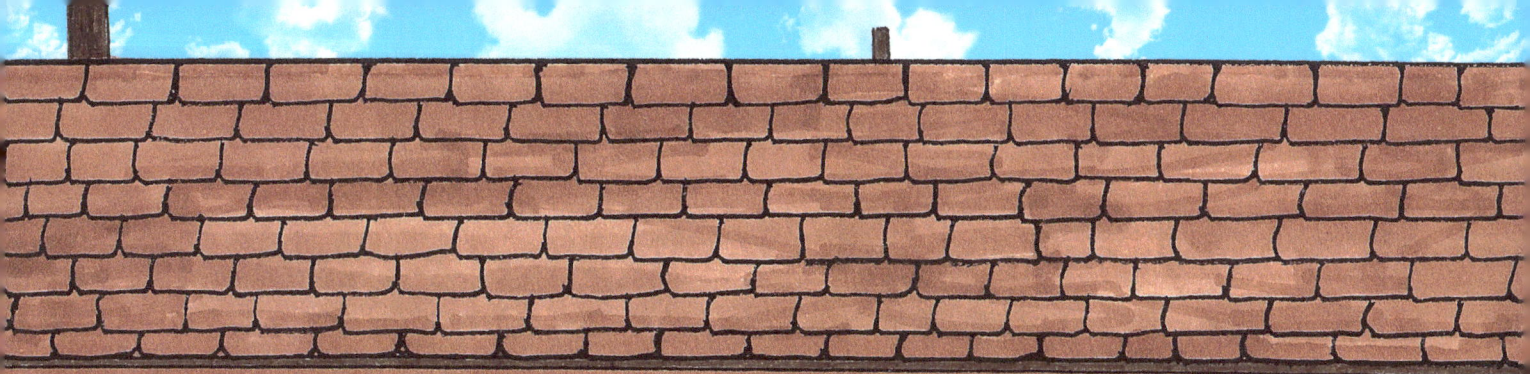

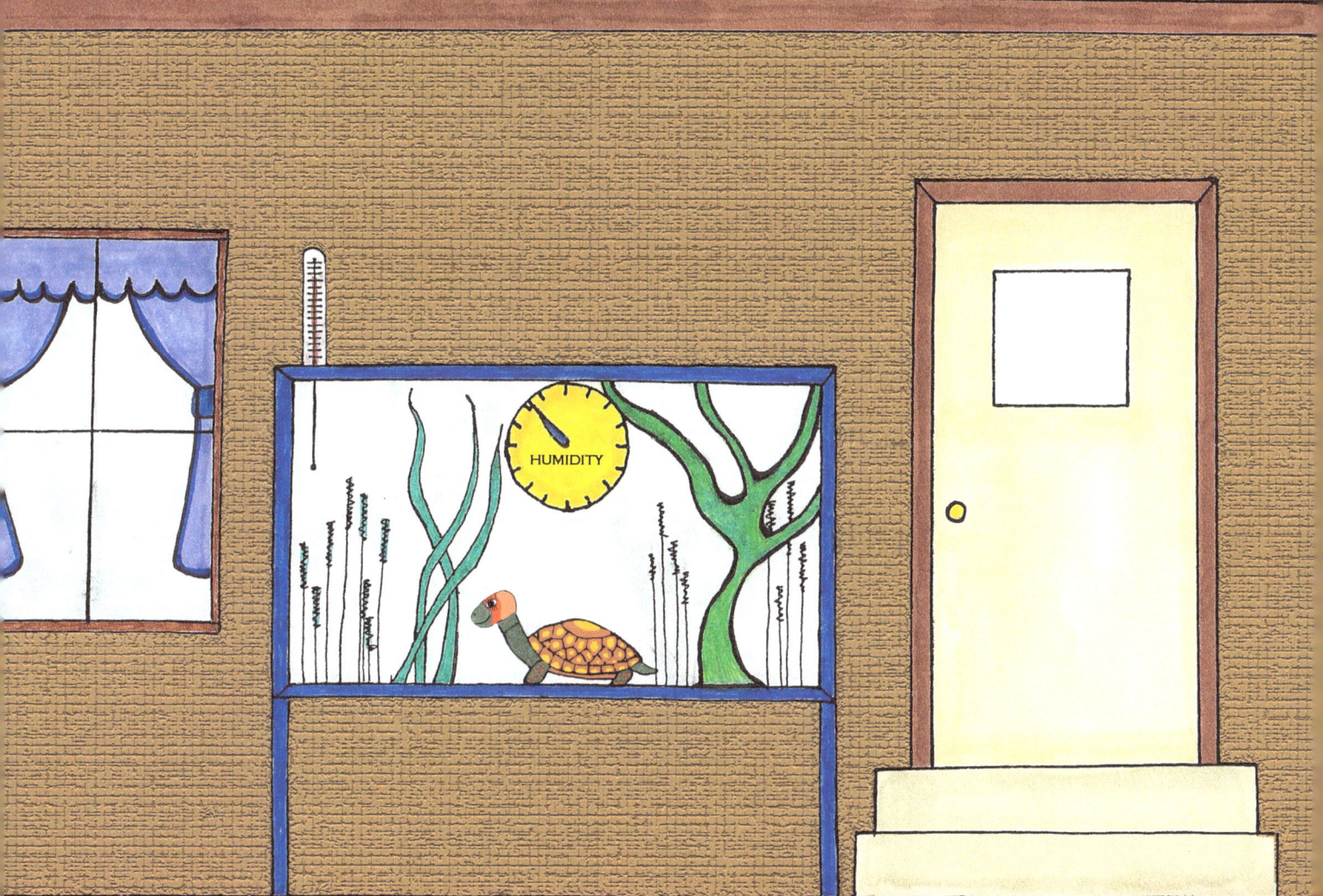

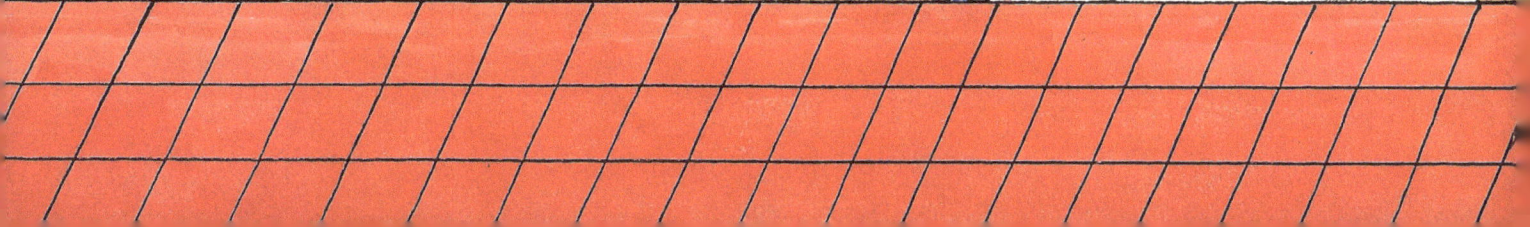

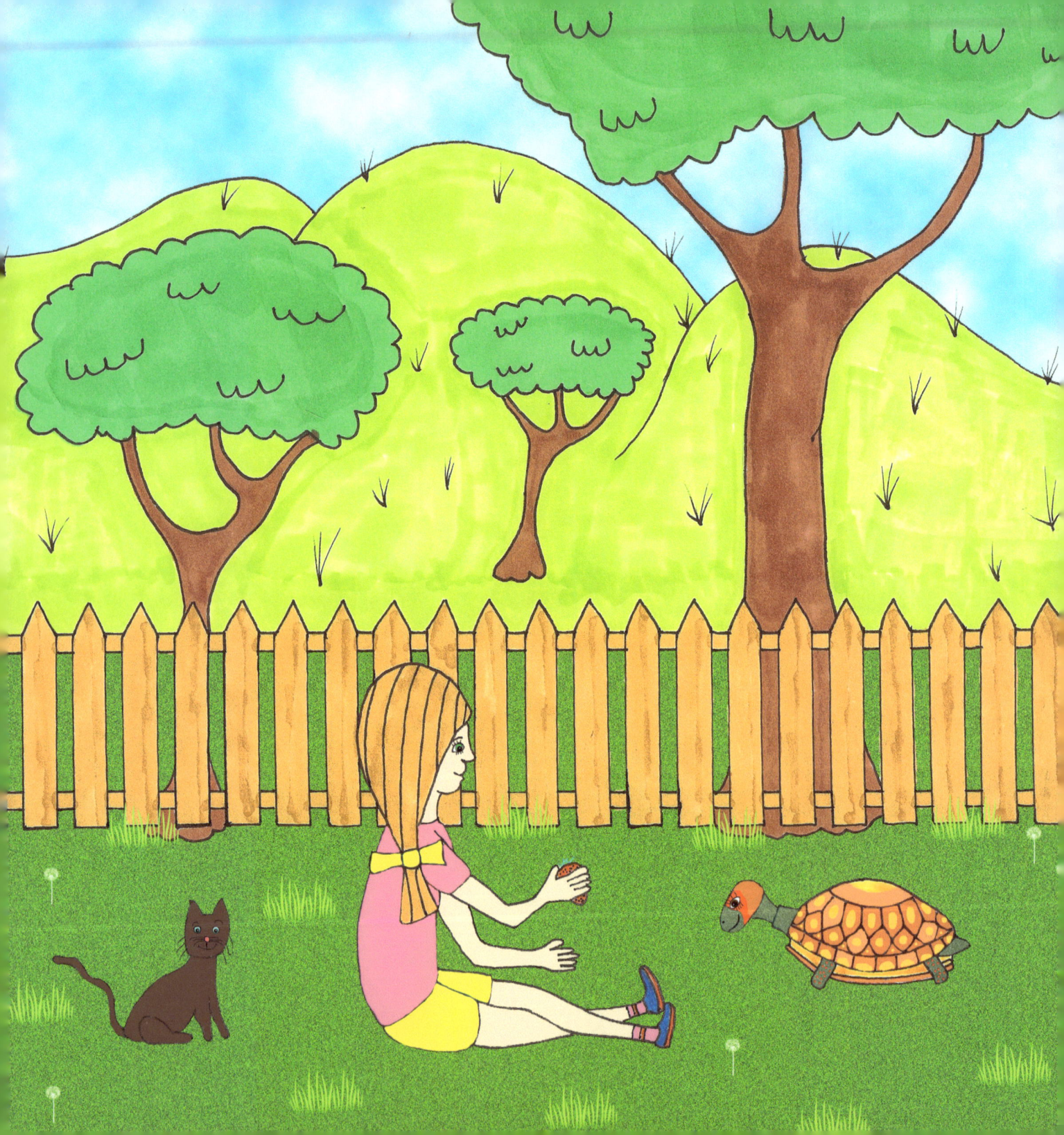

Mavis is an omnivore. This means she eats plants and animals. She likes worms, fresh veggies, mixed greens, and dandelion. She also takes calcium. On special occasions, I give her strawberries. Those are her favorite!

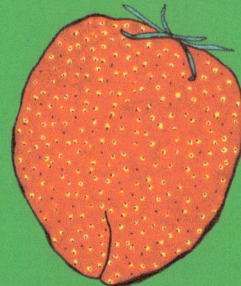

After we brought Mavis home, she got sick again. We had to take her back to see the veterinarian at the Reptile Rescue Center to find out what was wrong.

REPTILE RESCUE CENTER

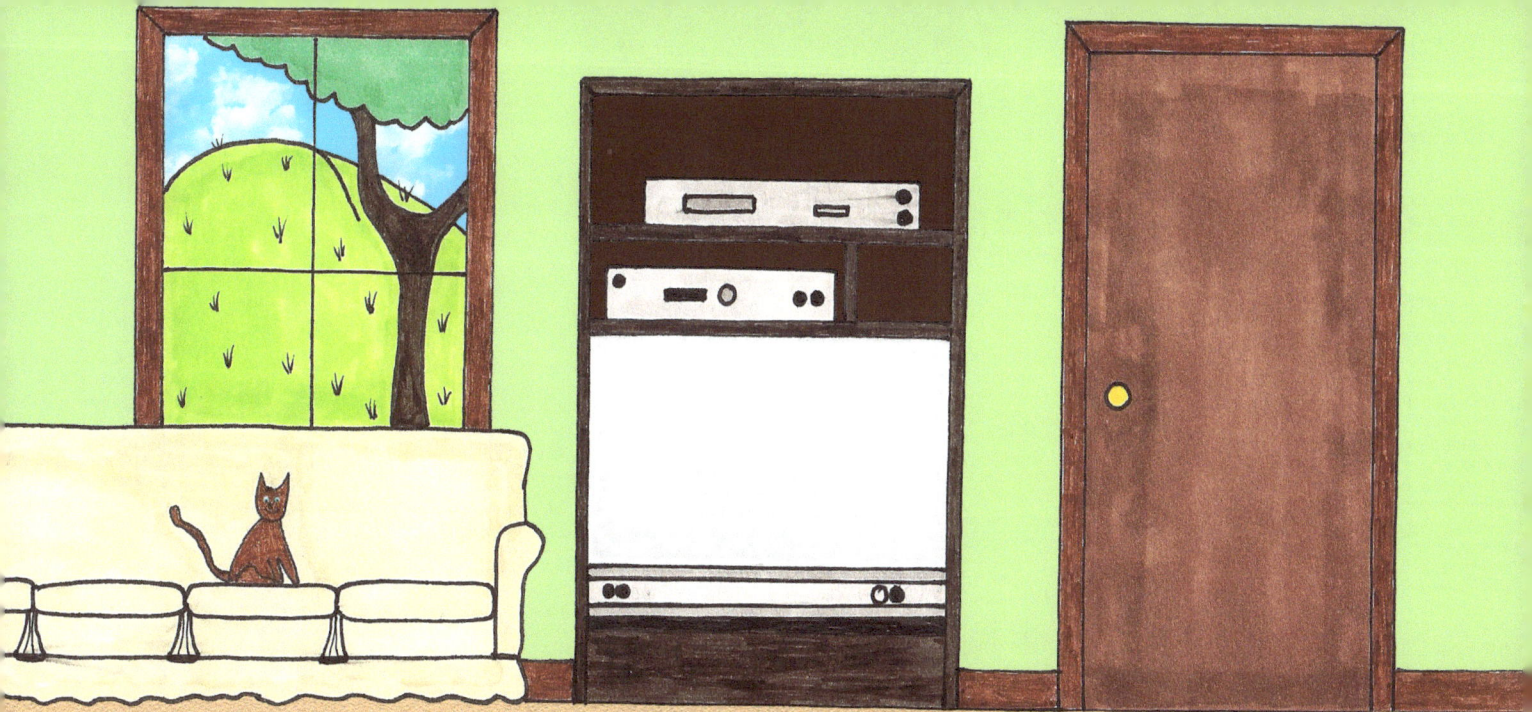

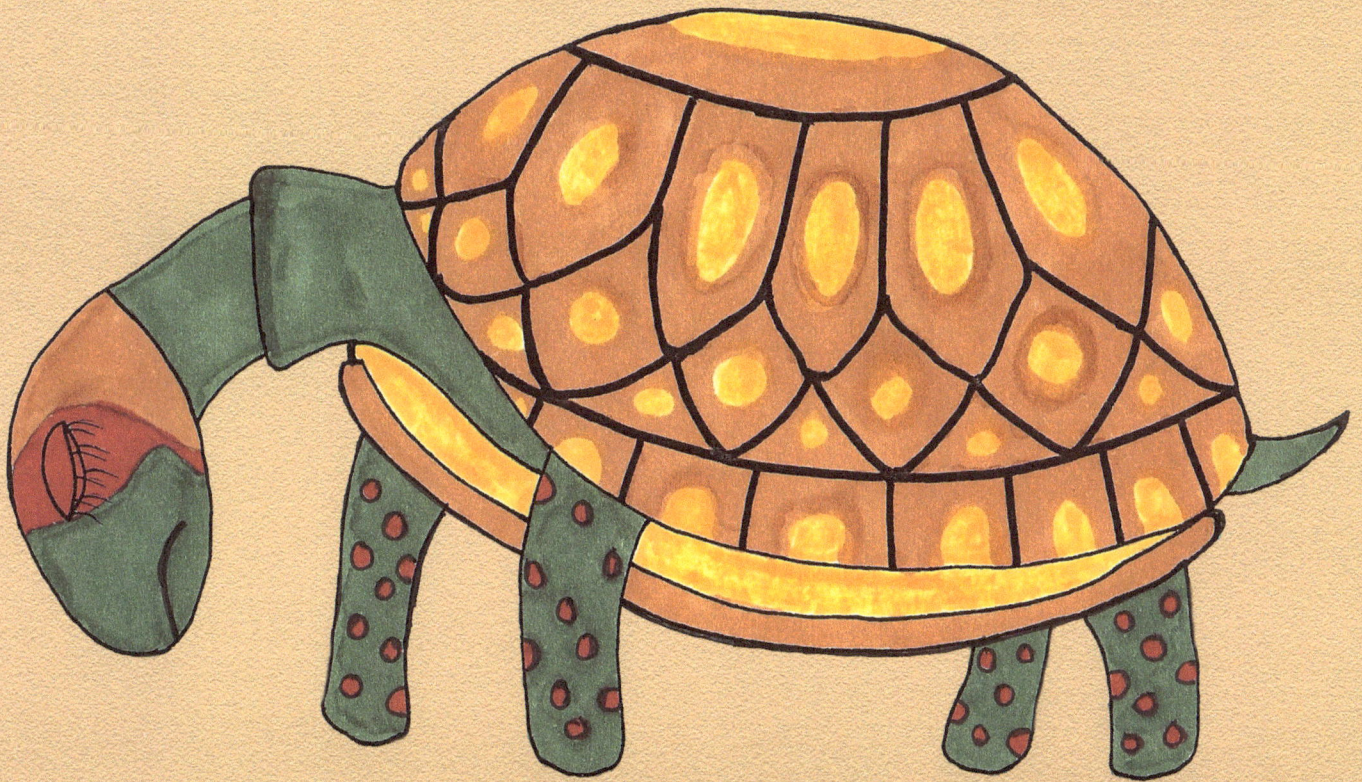

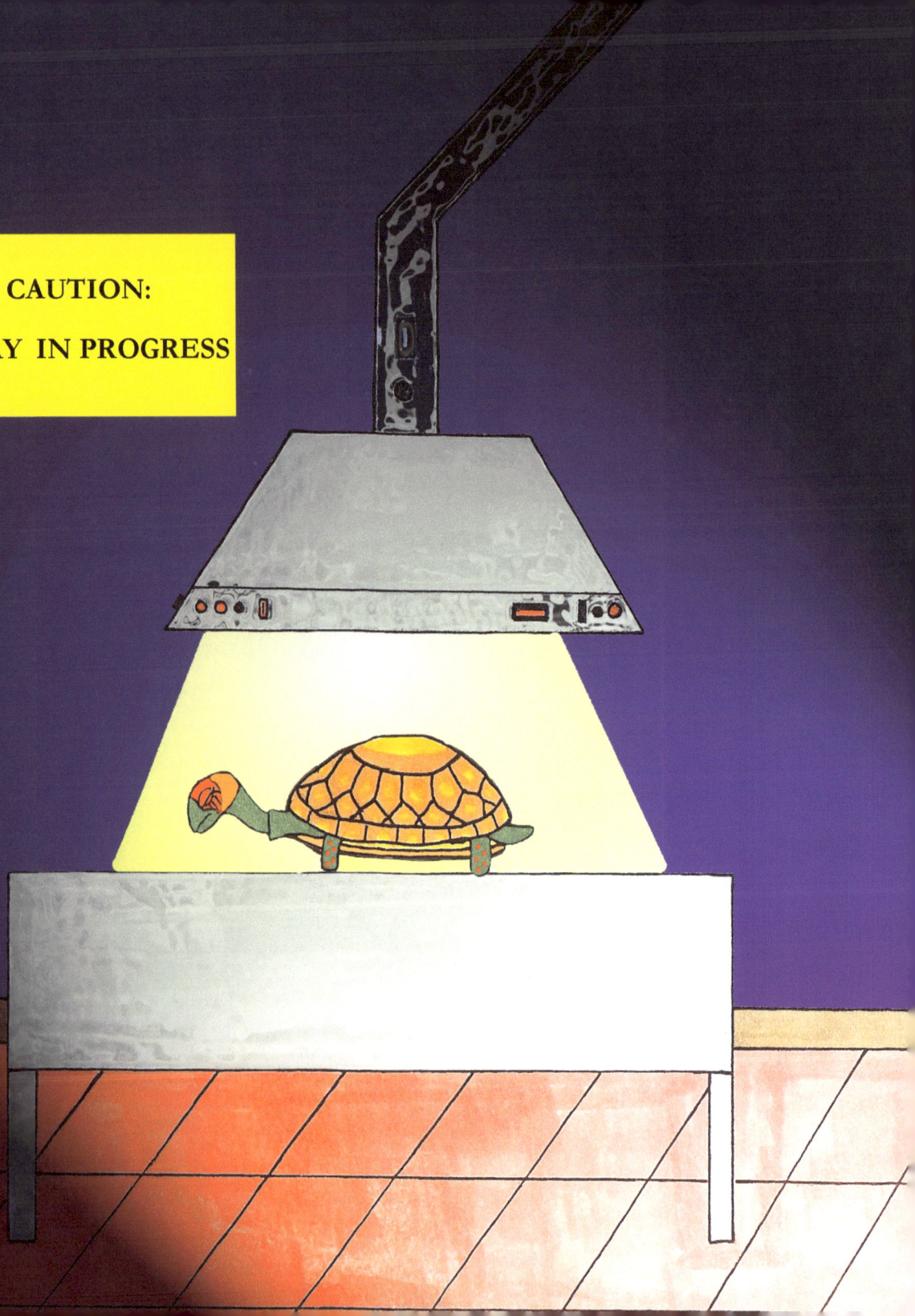

CAUTION:

X-RAY IN PROGRESS

The vet took an x-ray of Mavis.

Do you know what he found?

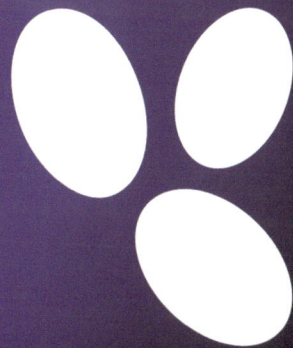

Eggs! Mavis had eggs inside of her that were stuck. This is called "egg binding". The shells were too soft for her to lay them.

The vet tried to help her pass the eggs, but it didn't work!

MAVIS X-RAY

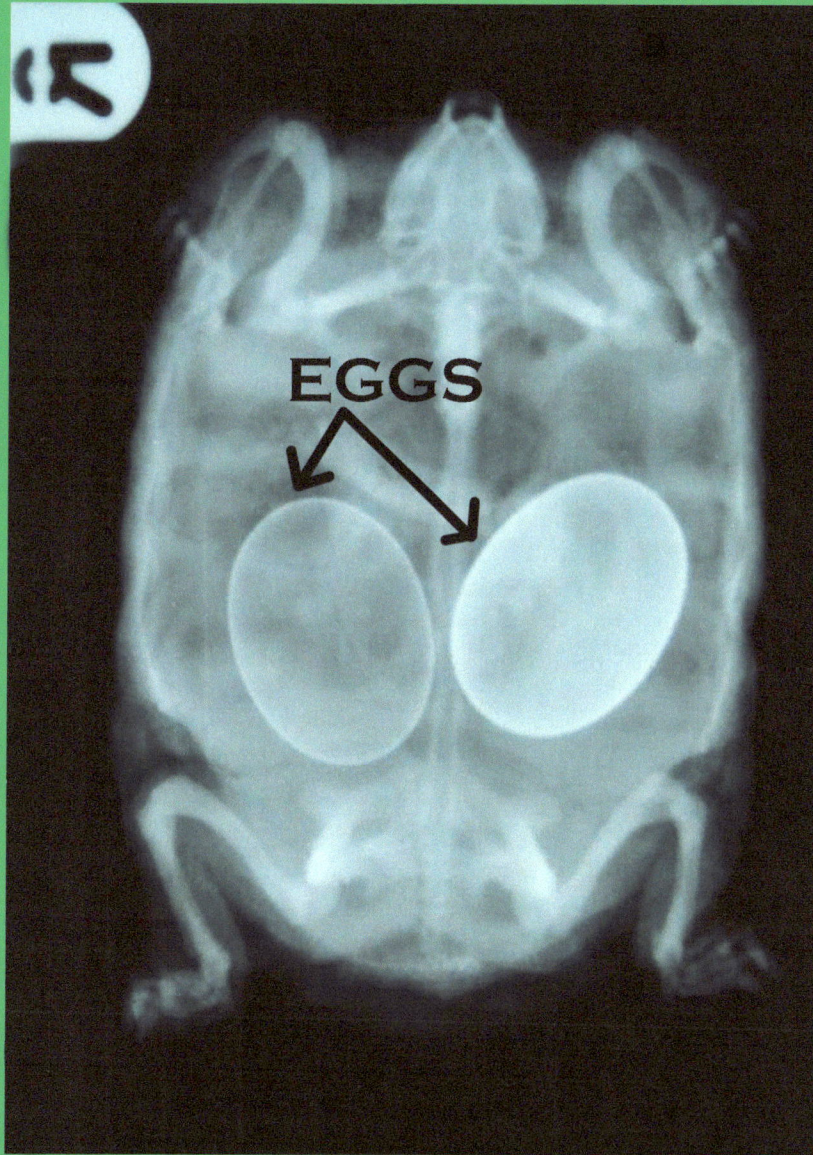

EGGS

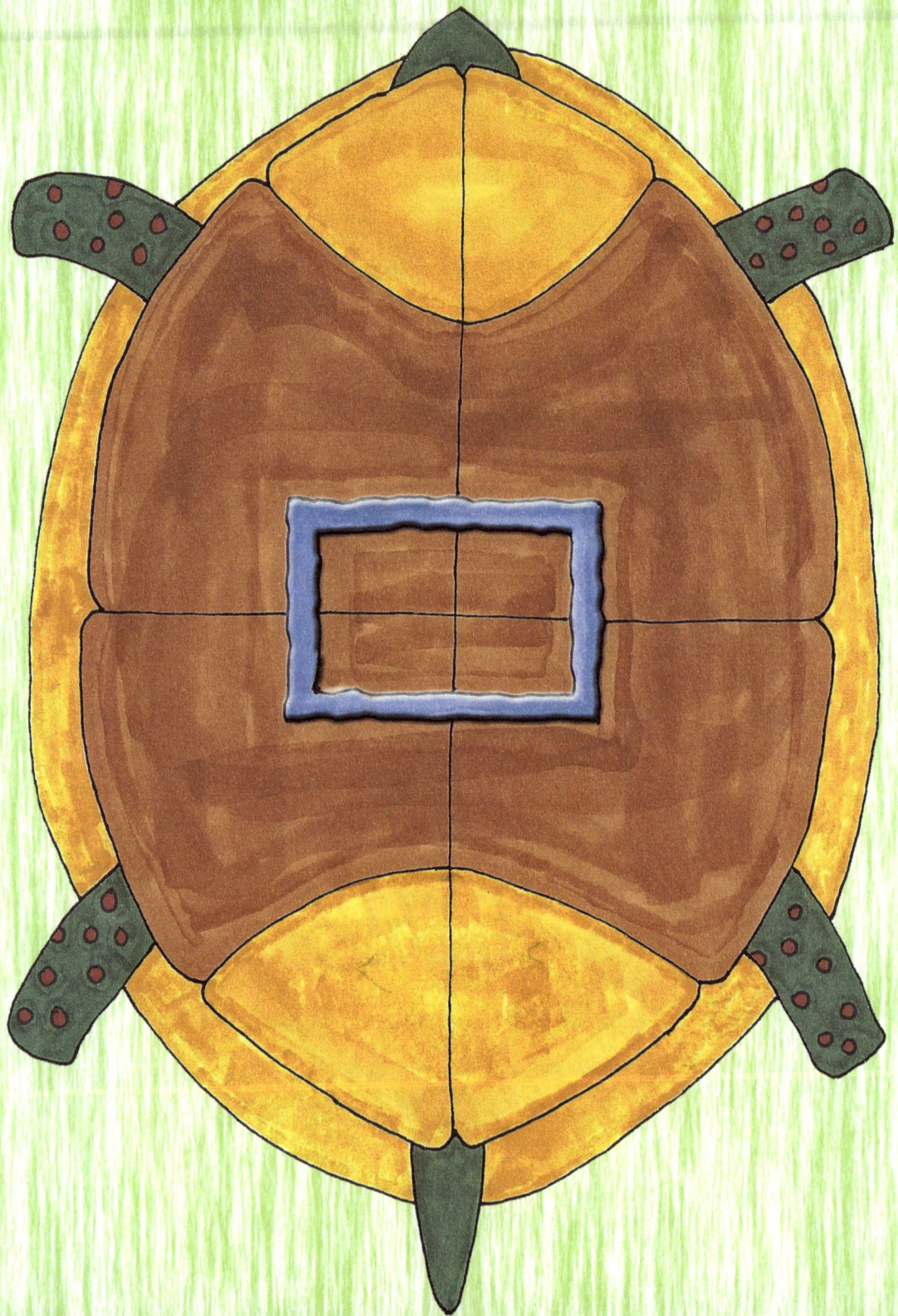

Mavis needed surgery to remove the bad eggs. They had to cut her plastron open to reach the eggs. The plastron is the bottom shell.

But don't worry, they repaired her shell with some special glue!

CHELONIAN SHELL
GLUE

Ingredients:
Polymethylmethacrylate

For Veterinary Use Only

Mavis is as good as new! She feels great and is back to eating and playing with her reptile friends!

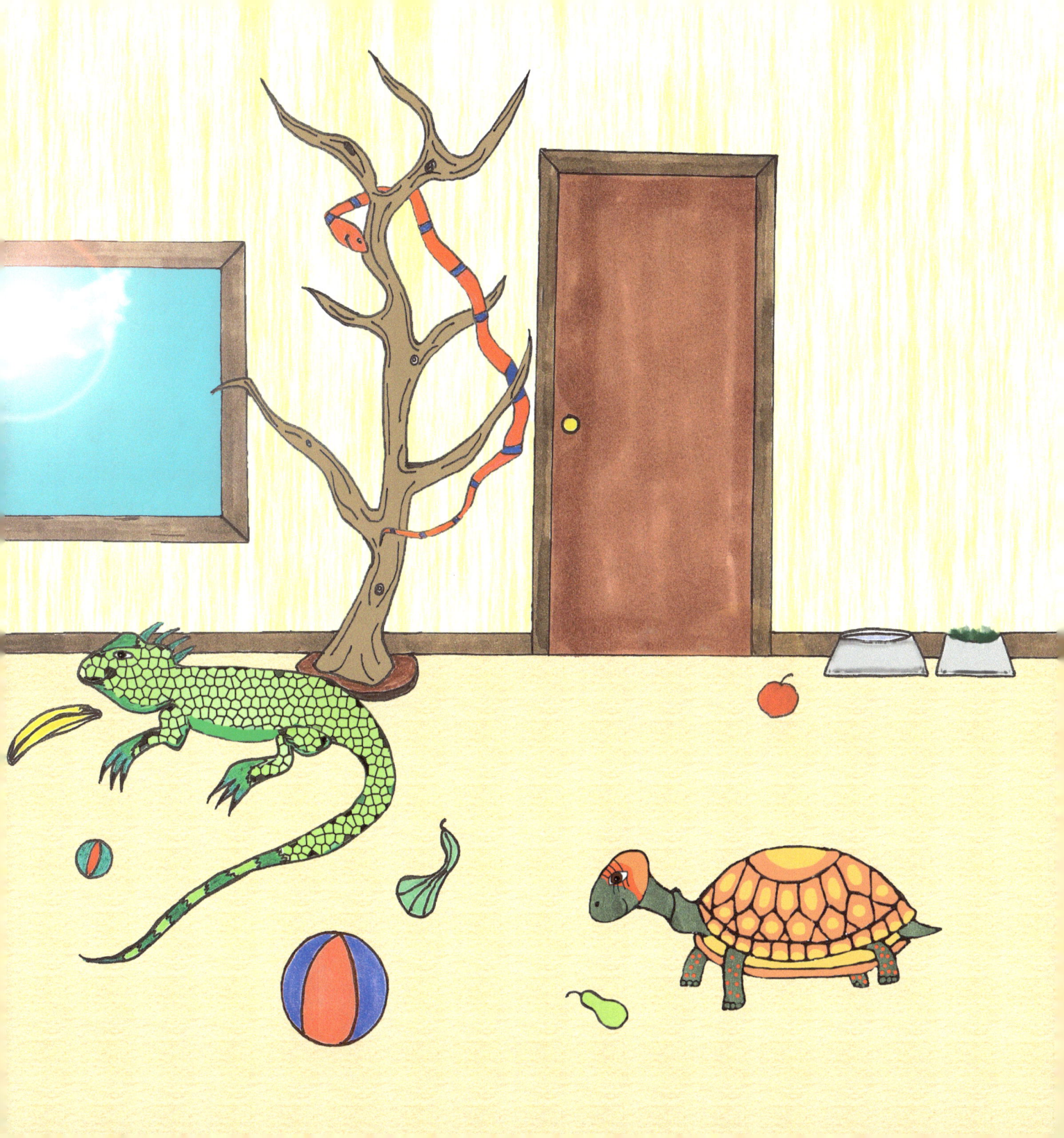

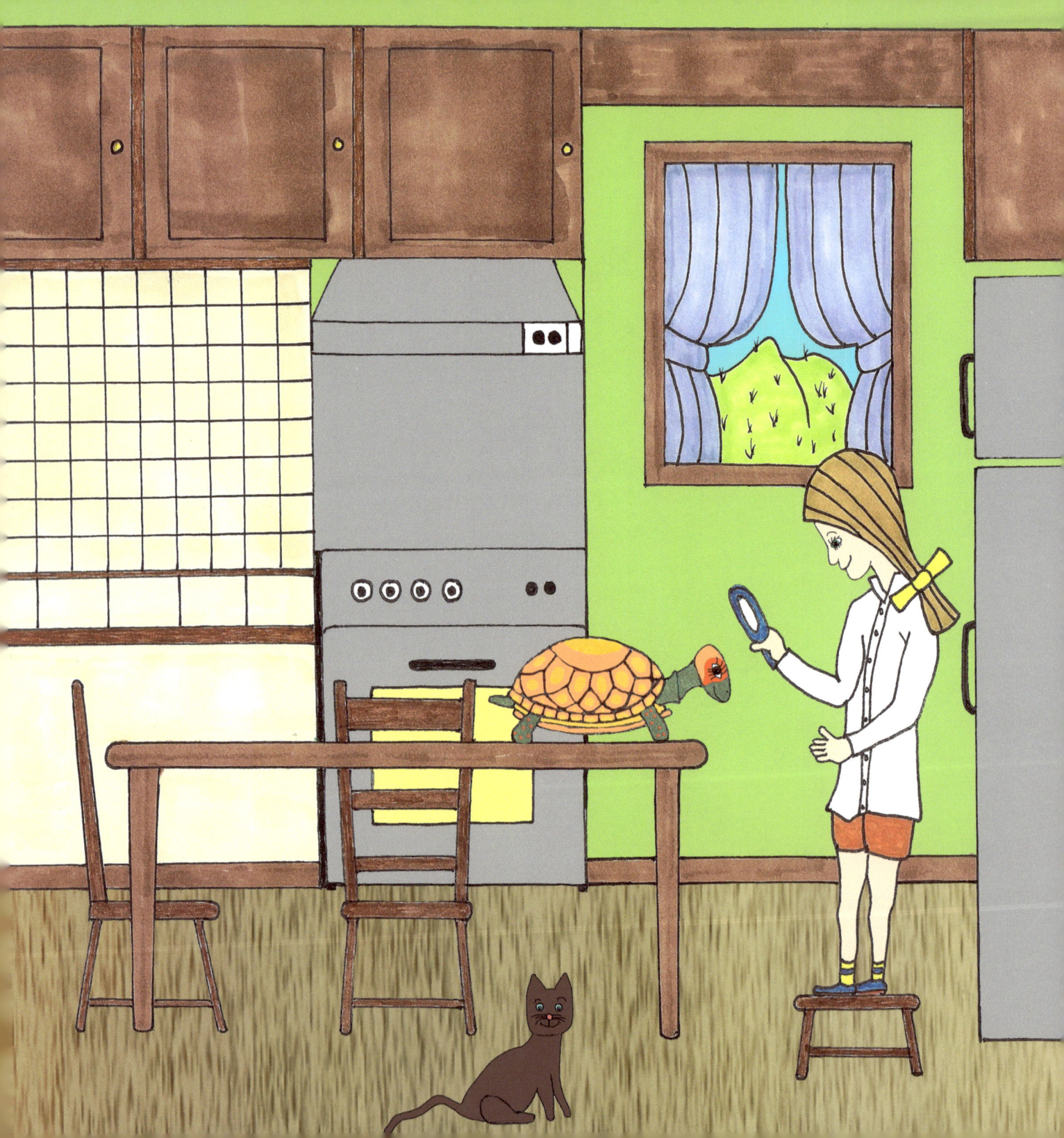

When I grow up, I want to be an exotics veterinarian so I can help unique creatures like Mavis when they are sick!

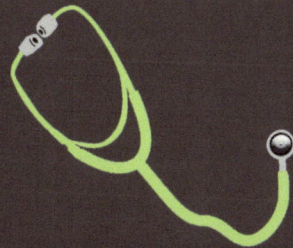

Glossary

Dehydrated- lacking water in the body from loss of bodily fluids, or from being deprived of water.

Exotic animal- an animal that is unusual or unique; striking and different .

Habitat- the conditions and environment in which an animal or plant lives.

Herpetologist- a scientist who studies reptiles and amphibians.

Omnivore- an animal that eats both plants and animals.

Plastron- the bottom portion of the shell of a turtle or tortoise. The top shell is called the carapace.

Reptiles- cold blooded creatures such as snakes, turtles, and lizards, which are covered in scales and lay eggs.

Terrarium- an enclosed land based habitat for pets meant for observation and to simulate the natural environment.

Tortoise- a member of the turtle family which lives on land; a slow moving reptile with a dome-shaped shell into which it can retract it's head and limbs. A turtle or tortoise is also called a chelonian.

Veterinarian- an animal doctor.

X-ray- a radiograph; a type of high energy radiation used to diagnose diseases by making pictures of the inside of the body.

About Little Vet™ Books
A note from the author:

Little Vet™ Books are designed for children with a desire to learn more about animals and veterinary medicine. Our books are written so that young readers may help the vet make a diagnosis, treat the pet, and see them get better. Little Vet™ Books also teach children about pet care, basic species knowledge, and introduce new medical terms. Perfect for little ones who love animals and want to be a vet when they grow up!

Please visit us at www.LittleVet.com to learn more about this series! Other available titles include:

Albert Einstein Goes to the Vet   **Razz Has Surgery**

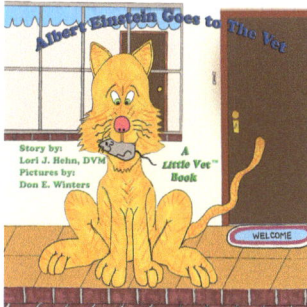

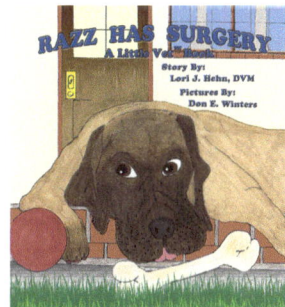

Thank you for reading Little Vet™ Books! We hope that your children have enjoyed the books in this series as much as we have enjoyed creating them!

www.ingramcontent.com/pod-product-compliance
Lightning Source LLC
Chambersburg PA
CBHW041236040426

42445CB00004B/49